Keto Air Fried Snack & Appetizer

Healthy Recipes for Better Snacks

Lydia Gorman

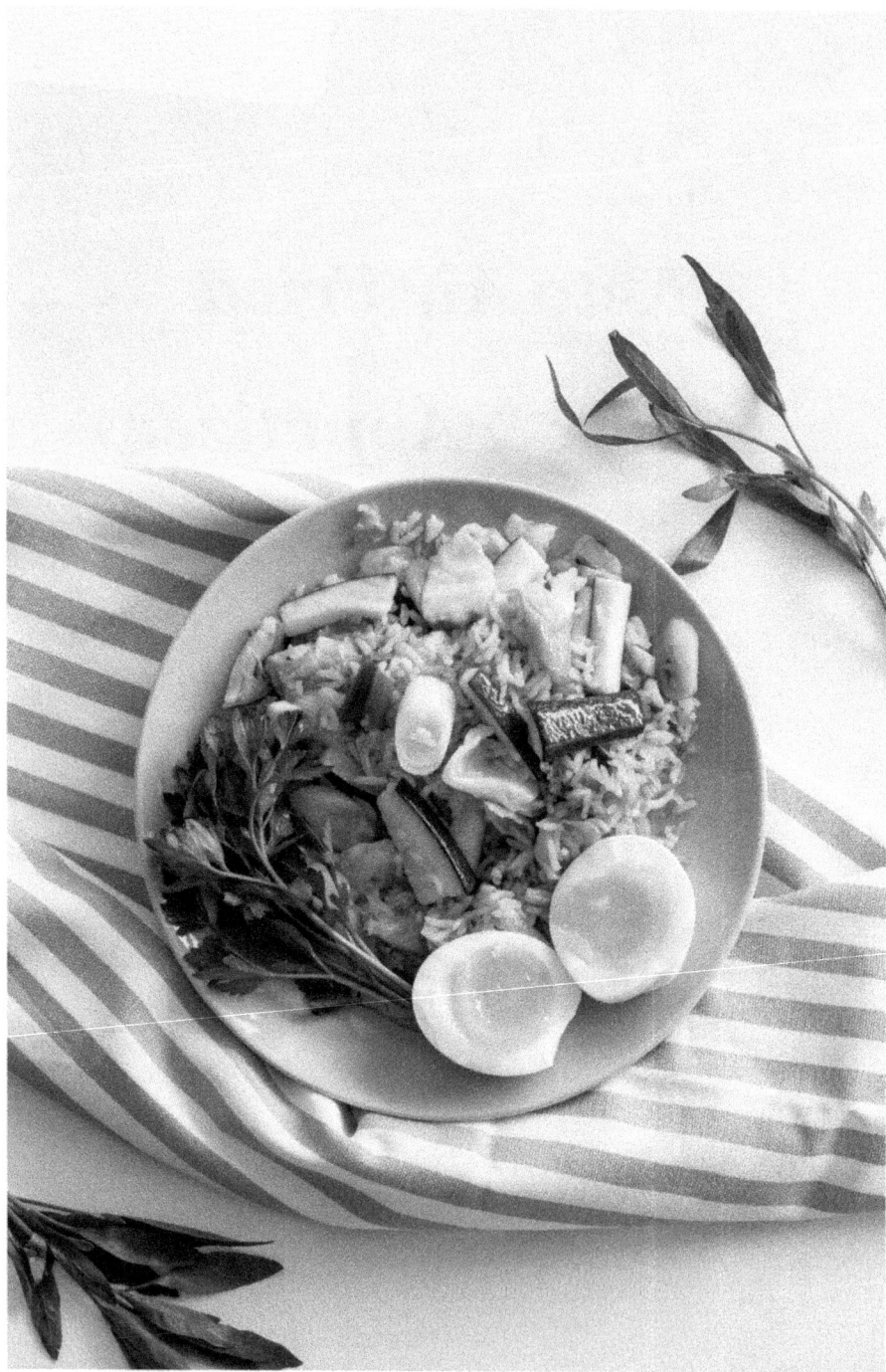

Table of Contents

Introduction

What's the difference between an air fryer and deep fryer? Air fryers bake food at a high temperature with a high-powered fan, while deep fryers cook food in a vat of oil that has been heated up to a specific temperature. Both cook food quickly, but an air fryer requires practically zero preheat time while a deep fryer can take upwards of 10 minutes. Air fryers also require little to no oil and deep fryers require a lot that absorb into the food. Food comes out crispy and juicy in both appliances, but don't taste the same, usually because deep fried foods are coated in batter that cook differently in an air fryer vs a deep fryer. Battered foods needs to be sprayed with oil before cooking in an air fryer to help them color and get crispy, while the hot oil soaks into the batter in a deep fryer. Flour-based batters and wet batters don't cook well in an air fryer, but they come out very well in a deep fryer.

The ketogenic diet is one such example. The diet calls for a very small number of carbs to be eaten. This means food such as rice, pasta, and other starchy vegetables like potatoes are off the menu. Even relaxed versions of the keto diet minimize carbs to a large extent and this compromises the goals of many dieters. They end up having to exert large amounts of willpower to follow the diet. This doesn't do them any favors since willpower is like a muscle. At some point, it tires and this is when the dieter goes right back to their old pattern of eating. I have personal experience with this. In terms of health benefits, the keto diet offers the most. The reduction of carbs forces your body to mobilize fat and this results in automatic fat loss and better health.

Feel free to mix and match the recipes you see in here and play around with them. Eating is supposed to be fun! Unfortunately, we've associated fun eating with unhealthy food. This doesn't have to be the case. The air fryer, combined with the Mediterranean diet, will make your mealtimes fun-filled again and full of taste. There's no grease and messy cleanups to deal with anymore. Are you excited yet?

You should be! You're about to embark on a journey full of air fried goodness!

Cauliflower Hummus

Preparation Time: 10 minutes

Cooking Time: 35 minutes

Serve: 8

Ingredients:

1 cauliflower head, cut into florets

3 tbsp olive oil

1/2 tsp ground cumin

1 tsp garlic, chopped

2 tbsp fresh lemon juice

1/3 cup tahini

Pepper

Salt

Directions:

Place the cooking tray in the air fryer basket.

Line air fryer basket with parchment paper.

Select Bake mode.

Set time to 35 minutes and temperature 400 F then press START.

The air fryer display will prompt you to ADD FOOD once the temperature is reached then spread cauliflower onto the parchment paper in the air fryer basket.

roasted cauliflower into the food processor along with remaining ingredients and process until smooth.

Serve and enjoy

Spicy Mixed Nuts

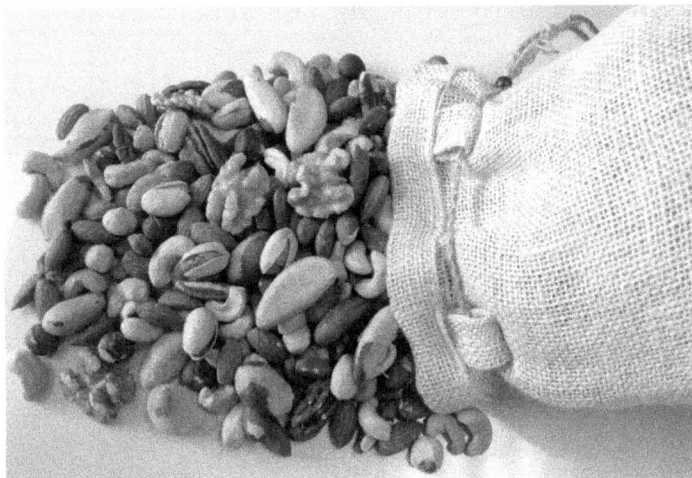

Preparation Time: 10 minutes

Cooking Time: 4 minutes

Serve: 2

Ingredients:

2 cup mixed nuts

1 tsp chili powder

1 tsp ground cumin

1 tbsp olive oil

1 tsp pepper

1 tsp salt

Directions:

In a bowl, add all ingredients and toss well.

Place the cooking tray in the air fryer basket.

Line air fryer basket with parchment paper.

Select Air Fry mode.

Set time to 4 minutes and temperature 350 F then press START.

The air fryer display will prompt you to ADD FOOD once the temperature is reached then place mixed nuts onto the parchment paper in the air fryer basket. Serve and enjoy.

Tasty Cauliflower Bites

Preparation Time: 10 minutes

Cooking Time: 15 minutes

Serve: 4

Ingredients:

1 lb cauliflower florets

1/2 tsp dried rosemary

1 1/2 tsp garlic powder

1 tbsp olive oil

1 tsp sesame seeds

1 tsp ground coriander

Pepper

Salt

Directions:

Place the cooking tray in the air fryer basket.

Line air fryer basket with parchment paper.

Select Bake mode.

Set time to 15 minutes and temperature 400 F then press START.

The air fryer display will prompt you to ADD FOOD once the temperature is reached then spread cauliflower florets onto the parchment paper in the air fryer basket. Serve and enjoy.

Crab Dip

Preparation Time: 10 minutes

Cooking Time: 7 minutes

Serve: 4

Ingredients:

1 cup crab, cooked

2 tbsp fresh parsley, chopped

2 tbsp fresh lemon juice

2 tbsp hot sauce

2 cups Jalapeno jack cheese, grated

1/2 cup green onions, sliced

1/4 cup mayonnaise

1 tsp pepper

1/2 tsp salt

Directions:

Add all ingredients except parsley and lemon juice in the 6-inch baking dish and mix well.

Select Air Fry mode.

Set time to 7 minutes and temperature 400 F then press START.

The air fryer display will prompt you to ADD FOOD once the temperature is reached then place the baking dish in the air fryer basket.

Remove dish from air fryer.

Add parsley and lemon juice.

Mix well. Serve and enjoy.

Broccoli Cheese Balls

Preparation Time: 10 minutes

Cooking Time: 30 minutes

Serve: 20

Ingredients:

2 eggs

1/4 cup onion, minced

1/2 cup almond flour

2 cups broccoli florets

1 tsp Italian seasoning

1 garlic clove, minced

1 cup cheddar cheese, shredded

Pepper

Salt

Directions:

Steam broccoli florets in boiling water until tender.

Drain well and chopped.

In a large bowl, mix together broccoli, eggs, cheese, almond flour, onion, garlic, and spices until well combined.

Make small balls from the mixture.

Place the cooking tray in the air fryer basket.

Line air fryer basket with parchment paper.

Select Bake mode.

Set time to 30 minutes and temperature 400 F then press START.

The air fryer display will prompt you to ADD FOOD once the temperature is reached then place broccoli balls onto the parchment paper in the air fryer basket.

Serve and enjoy.

Pepperoni Chips

Preparation Time: 10 minutes

Cooking Time: 10 minutes

Serve: 2

Ingredients:

1 oz pepperoni

4 tbsp mozzarella cheese, shredded

2 tbsp parmesan cheese, grated

1/2 tsp Italian seasoning

Directions:

Place the cooking tray in the air fryer basket.

Line air fryer basket with parchment paper.

Select Bake mode.

Set time to 10 minutes and temperature 400 F then press START.

The air fryer display will prompt you to ADD FOOD once the temperature is reached then arrange pepperoni onto the parchment paper in the air fryer basket.

Sprinkle parmesan cheese, Italian seasoning, and mozzarella cheese over pepperoni.

Serve and enjoy.

Simple Parmesan Zucchini Bites

Preparation Time: 10 minutes

Cooking Time: 15 minutes

Serve: 4

Ingredients:

1 egg

1/2 cup parmesan cheese, grated

2 cups zucchini, grated

1/4 cup cilantro, chopped

Pepper

Salt

Directions:

In a bowl, mix together zucchini, cilantro, cheese, egg, pepper, and salt.

Pour mixture into the small baking dish.

Select Bake mode.

Set time to 15 minutes and temperature 400 F then press START.

The air fryer display will prompt you to ADD FOOD once the temperature is reached then place the baking dish in the air fryer basket.

Serve and enjoy.

Yummy Chicken Dip

Preparation Time: 10 minutes

Cooking Time: 25 minutes

Serve: 6

Ingredients:

2 cups chicken, cooked and shredded

1/2 cup sour cream

8 oz cream cheese, softened

4 tbsp hot sauce

Directions:

Add all ingredients in a large bowl and mix until well combined.

Transfer mixture in a baking dish.

Cover dish with foil.

Select Bake mode.

Set time to 25 minutes and temperature 350 F then press START.

The air fryer display will prompt you to ADD FOOD once the temperature is reached then place the baking dish in the air fryer basket.

Serve and enjoy.

Roasted Cauliflower Florets

Preparation Time: 10 minutes

Cooking Time: 20 minutes

Serve: 4

Ingredients:

5 cups cauliflower florets

1/2 tsp cumin powder

1/2 tsp garlic powder 1

/4 tsp onion powder

1/4 tsp chili powder

1/2 tsp coriander powder

4 tablespoons olive oil

1/2 tsp salt

Directions:

Add all ingredients into the large bowl and toss well.

Place the cooking tray in the air fryer basket.

Line air fryer basket with parchment paper.

Select Air Fry mode.

Set time to 20 minutes and temperature 400 F then press START.

The air fryer display will prompt you to ADD FOOD once the temperature is reached then place cauliflower florets onto the parchment paper in the air fryer basket. Serve and enjoy.

Healthy Carrots Chips

Preparation Time: 10 minutes

Cooking Time: 12 minutes

Serve: 4

Ingredients:

12 oz carrot chips

1 tbsp olive oil

1/4 tsp paprika

1/4 tsp pepper

1/2 tsp garlic powder

1/2 tsp salt

Directions:

Add all ingredients into the bowl and toss well.

Place the cooking tray in the air fryer basket.

Line air fryer basket with parchment paper.

Select Air Fry mode.

Set time to 12 minutes and temperature 375 F then press START.

The air fryer display will prompt you to ADD FOOD once the temperature is reached then place carrot chips onto the parchment paper in the air fryer basket. Serve and enjoy.

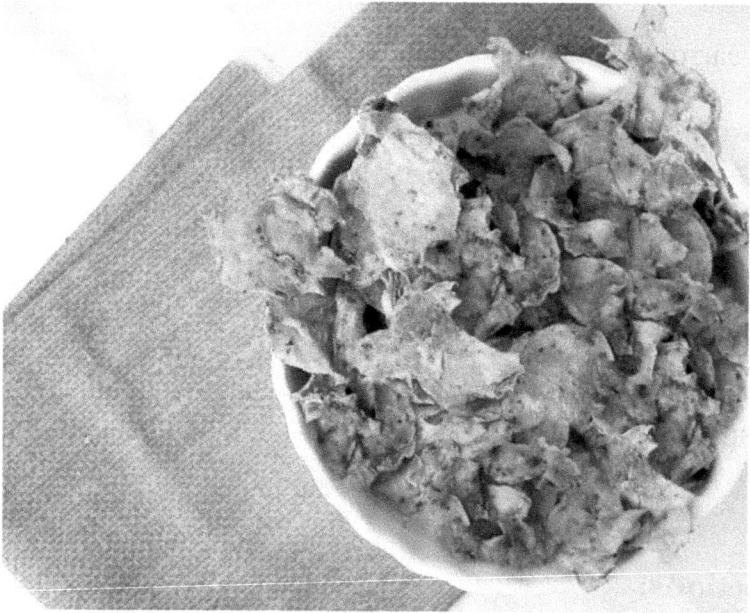

Herb Olives

Preparation Time: 10 minutes

Cooking Time: 5 minutes

Serve: 4

Ingredients:

2 cups olives

1/2 tsp crushed red pepper

2 tsp garlic, minced

2 tbsp olive oil

1/2 tsp dried fennel seeds

1/2 tsp dried oregano

Pepper

Salt

Directions:

Add olives and remaining ingredients into the mixing bowl and toss to coat well.

Place the cooking tray in the air fryer basket.

Line air fryer basket with parchment paper. Select Air Fry mode.

Set time to 5 minutes and temperature 300 F then press START.

The air fryer display will prompt you to ADD FOOD once the temperature is reached then place olives onto the parchment paper in the air fryer basket.

Serve and enjoy.

Healthy Mixed Nuts

Preparation Time: 5 minutes

Cooking Time: 20 minutes

Serve: 20

Ingredients:

5 cups mixed nuts

1 tsp paprika

1 tsp onion powder

1 tsp garlic powder

1/4 cup olive oil

1 tsp salt

Directions:

Add mixed nuts and remaining ingredients into the mixing bowl and mix well.

Place the cooking tray in the air fryer basket.

Line air fryer basket with parchment paper.

Select Bake mode.

Set time to 20 minutes and temperature 325 F then press START.

The air fryer display will prompt you to ADD FOOD once the temperature is reached then spread nuts onto the parchment paper in the air fryer basket.

Serve and enjoy.

Chicken Cheese Dip

Preparation Time: 10 minutes

Cooking Time: 10 minutes

Serve: 8

Ingredients:

2 cups cheddar cheese, shredded

1 cup ranch dressing

2 can chunk chicken, drained

1 package cream cheese

3/4 cup hot sauce

Directions:

Add chicken and hot sauce to the pan and cook for 2 minutes.

Add cream and ranch dressing and stir well.

Add half cheese and stir until well blended.

Transfer chicken mixture to the baking dish and sprinkle the remaining cheese on top.

Cover dish with foil.

Select Bake mode.

Set time to 10 minutes and temperature 370 F then press START.

The air fryer display will prompt you to ADD FOOD once the temperature is reached then place the baking dish in the air fryer basket.

 Serve and enjoy

Crispy Cauliflower Florets

Preparation Time: 10 minutes

Cooking Time: 15 minutes

Serve: 4

Ingredients:

1 medium cauliflower head, cut into florets

1/2 tsp Italian seasoning

1/4 tsp paprika

1/4 tsp onion powder

1 tbsp garlic, minced

3 tbsp olive oil

Pepper

Salt

Directions:

In a large bowl, toss cauliflower with remaining ingredients.

Place the cooking tray in the air fryer basket.

Line air fryer basket with parchment paper.

Select Bake mode.

Set time to 15 minutes and temperature 400 F then press START.

The air fryer display will prompt you to ADD FOOD once the temperature is reached then spread cauliflower florets onto the parchment paper in the air fryer basket. Serve and enjoy.

Goat Cheese Dip

Preparation Time: 10 minutes

Cooking Time: 10 minutes

Serve: 4

Ingredients:

10 oz goat cheese

2 garlic cloves, minced

1/4 tsp sage

1/4 tsp thyme

2 tbsp olive oil

1/4 cup parmesan cheese

Pepper

Salt

Directions:

Add all ingredients into the food processor and process until just combined.

Pour mixture into the prepared baking dish and spread well.

Select Bake mode.

Set time to 10 minutes and temperature 400 F then press START.

The air fryer display will prompt you to ADD FOOD once the temperature is reached then place the baking dish in the air fryer basket.

Serve and enjoy.

Mexican Cheese Dip

Preparation Time: 10 minutes

Cooking Time: 30 minutes

Serve: 10

Ingredients:

1/2 cup hot salsa

3 cups cheddar cheese, shredded

16 oz cream cheese, softened

1 cup sour cream

Directions:

In a bowl, mix together all ingredients until well combined and pour into the baking dish.

Cover dish with foil.

Select Bake mode.

Set time to 30 minutes and temperature 350 F then press START.

The air fryer display will prompt you to ADD FOOD once the temperature is reached then place the baking dish in the air fryer basket.

Serve and enjoy.

Air Fry Pecans

Preparation Time: 5 minutes

Cooking Time: 6 minutes

Serve: 6

Ingredients:

2 cups pecan halves

1 tbsp butter, melted

1/4 tsp chili powder

Salt

Directions:

Add pecans, chili powder, butter, and salt in a mixing bowl and toss well.

Place the cooking tray in the air fryer basket.

Line air fryer basket with parchment paper.

Select Bake mode.

Set time to 6 minutes and temperature 400 F then press START.

The air fryer display will prompt you to ADD FOOD once the temperature is reached then place pecans onto the parchment paper in the air fryer basket.

Serve and enjoy.

Stuffed Mushrooms

Preparation Time: 10 minutes

Cooking Time: 5 minutes

Serve: 3

Ingredients:

12 baby mushrooms

4 bacon slices, cooked and crumbled

4 oz cream cheese

2 tbsp butter, melted

Pepper

Salt

Directions:

In a small bowl, mix together cream cheese, butter, bacon, pepper, and salt.

Stuff cream cheese mixture into the mushrooms.

Place the cooking tray in the air fryer basket.

Line air fryer basket with parchment paper.

Select Bake mode.

Set time to 5 minutes and temperature 350 F then press START.

The air fryer display will prompt you to ADD FOOD once the temperature is reached then place stuffed mushrooms onto the parchment paper in the air fryer basket.

Serve and enjoy.

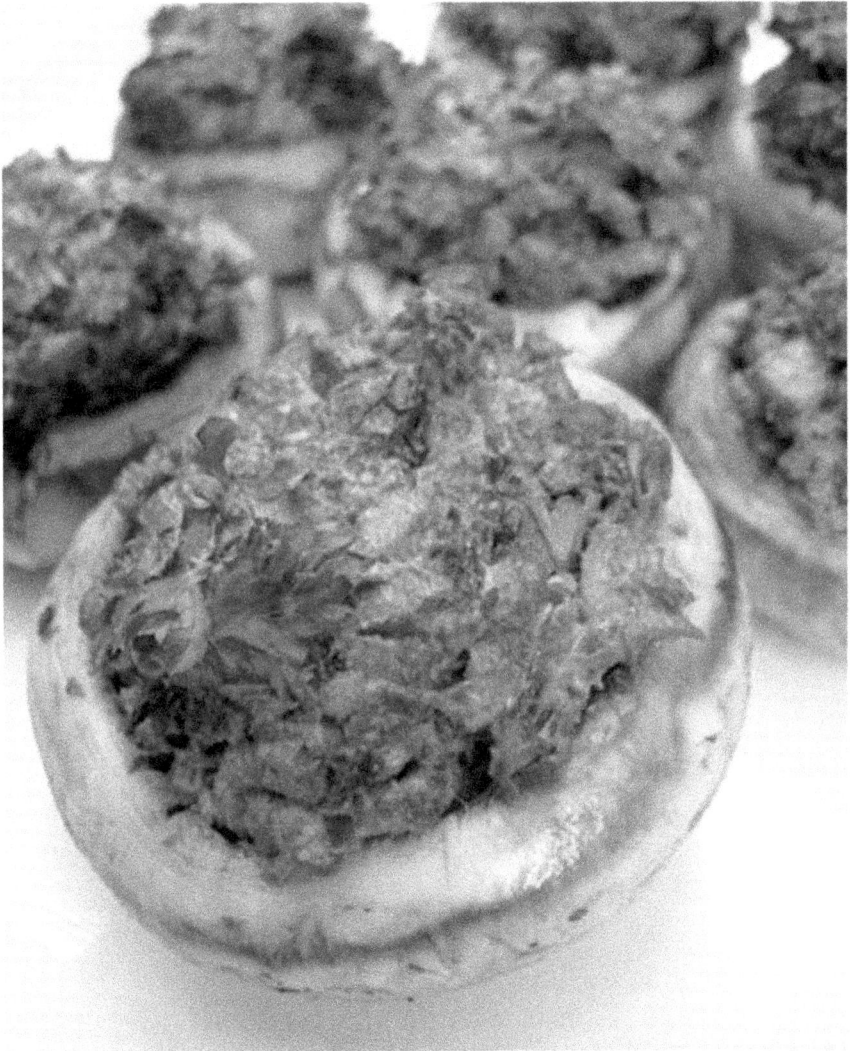

Roasted Nuts

Preparation Time: 10 minutes

Cooking Time: 15 minutes

Serve: 6

Ingredients:

1 cup cashew nuts

1 cup almonds

1/2 tsp chili powder

1 tbsp olive oil

1/2 tsp salt

Directions

In a bowl, toss almonds and cashew with oil, chili powder, and salt.

Place the cooking tray in the air fryer basket.

Line air fryer basket with parchment paper.

Select Bake mode.

Set time to 15 minutes and temperature 300 F then press START.

The air fryer display will prompt you to ADD FOOD once the temperature is reached then place cashew and almonds onto the parchment paper in the air fryer basket.

Serve and enjoy.

Cheese Pesto Jalapeno Poppers

Preparation Time: 10 minutes

Cooking Time: 15 minutes

Serve: 6

Ingredients:

3 jalapeno peppers, halved and remove seeds

3 tbsp basil pesto

1/4 cup cream cheese

1/2 cup mozzarella cheese, shredded

Directions:

In a bowl, mix together pesto, shredded cheese, and cream cheese.

Stuff pesto cheese mixture into each jalapeno half.

Place the cooking tray in the air fryer basket.

Line air fryer basket with parchment paper.

Select Bake mode.

Set time to 15 minutes and temperature 400 F then press START.

The air fryer display will prompt you to ADD FOOD once the temperature is reached then place stuffed jalapeno halves onto the parchment paper in the air fryer basket.

Serve and enjoy.

Italian-Style Tomato Chips

Prep + Cook Time: 20 minutes

2 Servings

INGREDIENTS

2 tomatoes, cut into thick rounds

1 teaspoon extra-virgin olive oil

Sea salt and fresh ground pepper, to taste

1 teaspoon Italian seasoning mix

¼ cup Romano cheese, grated

DIRECTIONS

Preheat air fryer to 350 F.

Toss the tomato sounds with remaining ingredients.

Transfer the tomato rounds to the cooking basket without overlapping.

Cook your tomato rounds in the preheated Air Fryer for 5 minutes.

Flip them over and cook an additional 5 minutes.

Work with batches. Serve warm.

Italian-Style Tomato-Parmesan Crisps

Prep + Cook Time: 20 minutes

4 Servings

INGREDIENTS

4 Roma tomatoes, sliced

2 tablespoons olive oil

Sea salt and white pepper, to taste

1 teaspoon Italian seasoning mix

4 tablespoons Parmesan cheese, grated

DIRECTIONS

Preheat air fryer to 350 F.

Generously grease the Air Fryer basket with nonstick cooking oil.

Toss the sliced tomatoes with the remaining ingredients.

Transfer them to the cooking basket without overlapping.

Cook in the preheated Air Fryer for 5 minutes.

Shake the cooking basket and cook an additional 5 minutes.

Work in batches.

Serve with Mediterranean aioli for dipping, if desired.

Enjoy!

Bruschetta with Fresh Tomato and Basil

Prep + Cook Time: 15 minutes

3 Servings

INGREDIENTS

½ Italian bread, sliced

2 garlic cloves, peeled

2 tablespoons extra-virgin olive oil

2 ripe tomatoes, chopped

1 teaspoon dried oregano

Salt, to taste

8 fresh basil leaves, roughly chopped

DIRECTIONS

Place the bread slices on the lightly greased Air Fryer grill pan.

Bake at 370 degrees F for 3 minutes.

Cut a clove of garlic in half and rub over one side of the toast; brush with olive oil.

Add the chopped tomatoes.

Sprinkle with oregano and salt.

Increase the temperature to 380 degrees F.

Cook in the preheated Air Fryer for 3 minutes more.

Garnish with fresh basil and serve. Serve and enjoy!

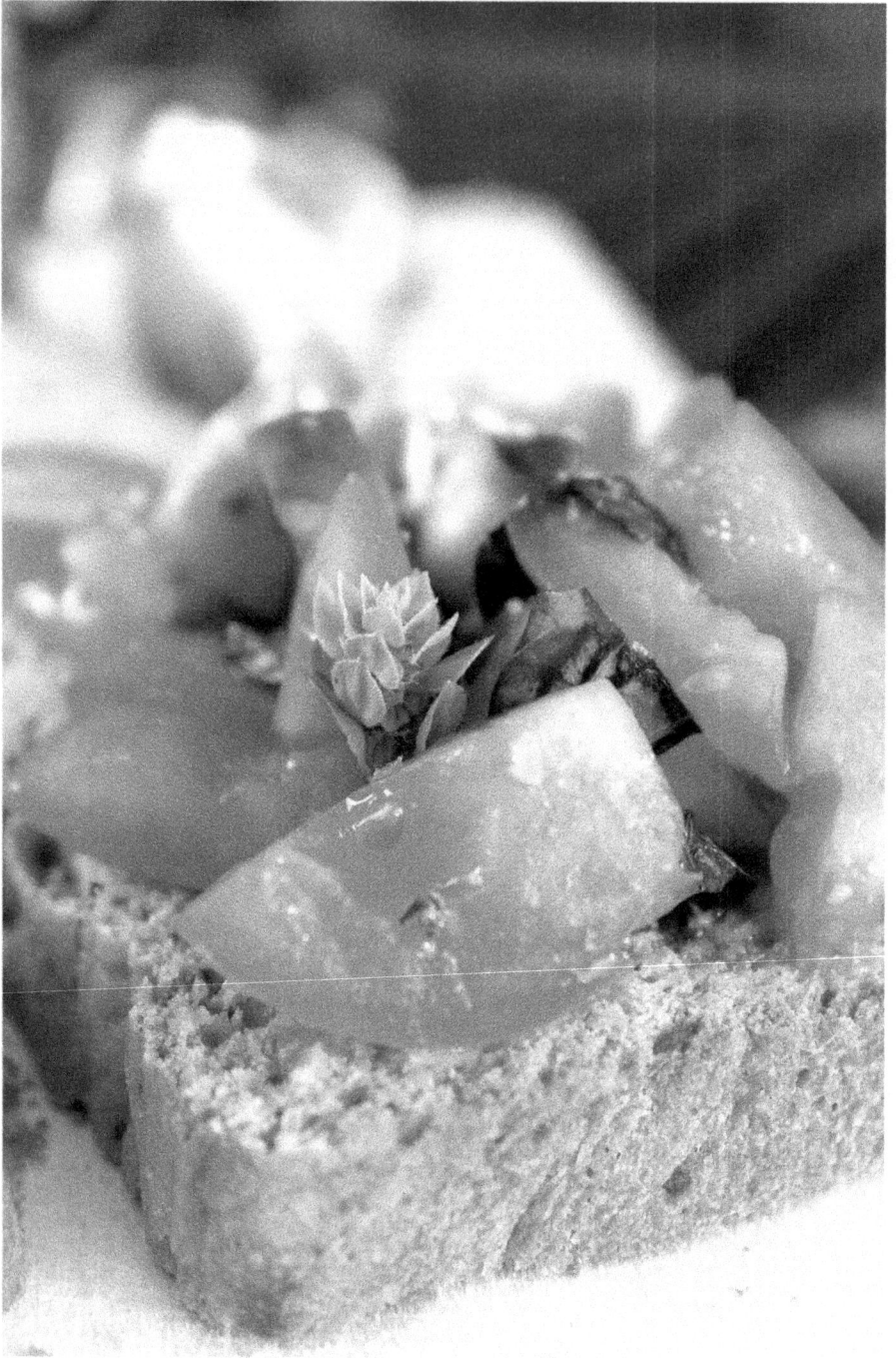

Root Vegetable Chips with Dill Mayonnaise

Prep + Cook Time: 40 minutes

4 Servings

INGREDIENTS

½ pound red beetroot, julienned

½ pound golden beetroot, julienned

¼ pound carrot, julienned

Sea salt and ground black pepper, to taste

1 teaspoon olive oil

½ cup mayonnaise

1 teaspoon garlic, minced

¼ teaspoon dried dill weed

DIRECTIONS

Toss your veggies with salt, black pepper and olive oil.

Arrange the veggie chips in a single layer in the Air Fryer cooking basket.

Cook the veggie chips in the preheated Air Fryer at 340 degrees F for 20 minutes; tossing the basket occasionally to ensure even cooking.

Work with two batches.

Meanwhile, mix the mayonnaise, garlic and dill until well combined.

Serve the vegetable chips with the mayo sauce on the side and serve.

Greek-Style Zucchini Rounds

Prep + Cook Time: 15 minutes

3 Servings

INGREDIENTS

½ pound zucchini, cut into thin rounds

1 teaspoon extra-virgin olive oil

½ teaspoon dried sage, crushed

½ teaspoon oregano

¼ teaspoon ground bay leaf

Coarse sea salt and ground black pepper, to taste

Greek dipping sauce:

½ cup Greek yogurt

½ teaspoon fresh lemon juice

2 tablespoons mayonnaise

½ teaspoon garlic, pressed

DIRECTIONS

Toss the zucchini rounds with olive oil and spices and place them in the Air Fryer cooking basket.

Cook in the preheated Air Fryer at 400 degrees F for 10 minutes; shaking the basket halfway through the cooking time.

Let it cool slightly and cook an additional minute or so until crispy and golden brown.

Meanwhile, make the sauce by whisking all the sauce ingredients; place the sauce in the refrigerator until ready to serve.

Serve the crispy zucchini rounds with Greek dipping sauce on the side.

Serve warm.

Crunchy Wontons with Sausage and Peppers

Prep + Cook Time: 20 minutes

3 Servings

INGREDIENTS

20 3-½-inch wonton wrappers

½ pound beef sausage crumbled

1 bell pepper, deveined and chopped

1 teaspoon sesame oil

½ teaspoon granulated garlic

1 tablespoon soy sauce

1 tablespoon rice wine vinegar

1 tablespoon honey

1 teaspoon Sriracha sauce

1 teaspoon sesame seeds, toasted

DIRECTIONS

Mix the crumbled sausage with the chopped pepper and set it aside.

Place wonton wrappers on a clean work surface.

Divide the sausage filling between the wrappers.

Wet the edge of each wrapper with water, fold the top half over the bottom half and pinch the border to seal.

Place the wontons in the cooking basket and brush them with a little bit of olive oil.

Cook the wontons at 400 degrees F for 8 minutes.

Work with batches.

In the meantime, whisk the sauce ingredients and set it aside.

Serve the warm wontons with the sauce for dipping.

Enjoy!

Sweet Potato Chips with Chili Mayo

Prep + Cook Time: 35 minutes

3 Servings

INGREDIENTS

1 sweet potato, cut into

1/8-inch-thick slices

1 teaspoon olive oil

Sea salt and cracked mixed peppercorns, to taste

½ teaspoon turmeric powder

⅓ cup mayonnaise

1 teaspoon granulated garlic

½ teaspoon red chili flakes

DIRECTIONS

Toss the sweet potato slices with olive oil, salt, cracked peppercorns and turmeric powder.

Cook your sweet potatoes at 380 degrees F for 33 to 35 minutes, tossing the basket every 10 minutes to ensure even cooking.

Work with batches.

Meanwhile, mix the mayonnaise, garlic and red chili flakes to make the sauce.

The sweet potato chips will crisp up as it cools.

Serve the sweet potato chips with the chili mayo on the side.

Prosciutto Stuffed Jalapeños

Prep + Cook Time: 15 minutes

2 Servings

INGREDIENTS

8 fresh jalapeño peppers, deseeded and cut in half lengthwise

4 ounces Ricotta cheese, at room temperature

¼ teaspoon cayenne pepper

½ teaspoon granulated garlic

8 slices prosciutto, chopped

DIRECTIONS

Place the fresh jalapeño peppers on a clean surface.

Mix the remaining ingredients in a bowl; divide the filling between the jalapeño peppers.

Transfer the peppers to the Air Fryer cooking basket.

Cook the stuffed peppers at 400 degrees F for 15 minutes.

Serve and enjoy!

Hot Roasted Cauliflower Florets

Prep + Cook Time: 20 minutes

3 Servings

INGREDIENTS

½ cup plain flour

½ teaspoon shallot powder

1 teaspoon garlic powder

¼ teaspoon dried dill weed

½ teaspoon chipotle powder

Sea salt and ground black pepper, to taste

½ cup rice milk

2 tablespoons coconut oil, softened

1 pound cauliflower florets

DIRECTIONS

In a mixing bowl, thoroughly combine the flour, spices, rice milk and coconut oil.

Mix to combine well.

Coat the cauliflower florets with the batter and allow the excess batter to drip back into the bowl.

Cook the cauliflower florets at 400 degrees F for 12 minutes, shaking the basket once or twice to ensure even browning.

Serve with some extra hot sauce, if desired.

Enjoy!

Apple Chips with Walnuts

Prep + Cook Time: 35 minutes

2 Servings

INGREDIENTS

2 apples, peeled, cored and sliced

½ teaspoon ground cloves

1 teaspoon cinnamon

¼ cup walnuts

DIRECTIONS

Toss the apple slices with ground cloves and cinnamon.

Place the apple slices in the Air Fryer cooking basket and cook at 360 degrees F for 10 minutes or until crisp.

Reserve.

Then, toast the walnuts at 300 degrees F for 10 minutes; now, shake the basket and cook for another 10 minutes.

Chop the walnuts and scatter them over the apple slices and serve.

Easy Mexican Elote

Prep + Cook Time: 10 minutes

2 Servings

INGREDIENTS

2 ears of corn, husked

4 tablespoons Mexican crema

4 tablespoons Mexican cheese blend, crumbled

1 teaspoon fresh lime juice

Sea salt and chili powder, to taste

1 tablespoon fresh cilantro, chopped

DIRECTIONS

Cook the corn in the preheated Air Fryer at 390 degrees F for about 6 minutes.

Mix the Mexican crema, Mexican cheese blend, lime juice, salt and chili powder in a bowl.

Afterwards, insert a wooden stick into the core as a handle.

Rub each ear of corn with the topping mixture.

Garnish with fresh chopped cilantro.

Serve immediately.

Classic Jiaozi Chinese Dumplings

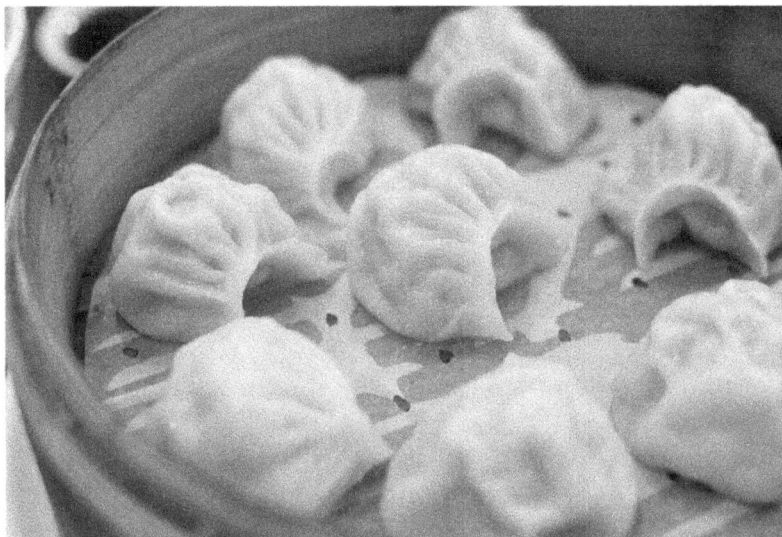

Prep + Cook Time: 15 minutes

3 Servings

INGREDIENTS

½ pound ground pork

1 cup Napa cabbage, shredded

2 scallion stalks, chopped

1 ounce bamboo shoots, shredded

½ teaspoon garlic paste

1 teaspoon fresh ginger, peeled and grated

8 ounces round wheat dumpling

Sauce:

2 tablespoons rice vinegar

¼ cup soy sauce

1 tablespoon ketchup

1 teaspoon deli mustard

1 teaspoon honey

1 teaspoon sesame seeds, lightly toasted

DIRECTIONS

Cook the pork in a wok that is preheated over medium-high heat; cook until no longer pink and stir in the Napa cabbage, scallions, bamboo shoots, garlic paste and ginger; salt to taste and stir to combine well.

Divide the pork mixture between dumplings.

Moisten the edge of each dumpling with water, fold the top half over the bottom half and press together firmly.

Place your dumplings in the Air Fryer cooking basket and spritz them with cooking spray.

Cook your dumplings at 400 degrees F for 8 minutes.

Work with batches.

While your dumplings are cooking, whisk the sauce ingredients.

Serve the warm dumplings with the sauce for dipping.

Enjoy!

Mexican-Style Corn on the Cob with Bacon

Prep + Cook Time: 20 minutes

3 Servings

INGREDIENTS

2 slices bacon

4 ears fresh corn, shucked and cut into halves

1 avocado, pitted, peeled and mashed

1 teaspoon ancho chili powder

2 garlic cloves

2 tablespoons cilantro, chopped

1 teaspoon lime juice

 Salt and black pepper, to taste

DIRECTIONS

Start by preheating your Air Fryer to 400 degrees F.

Cook the bacon for 6 to 7 minutes; chop into small chunks and reserve.

Spritz the corn with cooking spray.

Cook at 395 degrees F for 8 minutes, turning them over halfway through the cooking time.

Mix the reserved bacon with the remaining ingredients.

Spoon the bacon mixture over the corn on the cob and serve immediately.

Mini Plantain Cups

Prep + Cook Time: 10 minutes

3 Servings

INGREDIENTS

2 blackened plantains, chopped

¼ cup all-purpose flour

½ cup cornmeal

½ cup milk

1 tablespoon coconut oil

1 teaspoon fresh ginger, peeled and minced

A pinch of salt

A pinch of ground cinnamon

DIRECTIONS

In a mixing bowl, thoroughly combine all ingredients until everything is well incorporated.

Spoon the batter into a greased mini muffin tin.

Bake the mini plantain cups in your Air Fryer at 330 degrees F for 6 to 7 minutes or until golden brown.

Enjoy!

Sweet Potato Fries with Spicy Dip

Prep + Cook Time: 50 minutes

3 Servings

INGREDIENTS

3 medium sweet potatoes, cut into ⅓ -inch sticks

2 tablespoons olive oil

1 teaspoon kosher salt

Spicy Dip:

¼ cup mayonnaise

¼ cup Greek yogurt

¼ teaspoon Dijon mustard

1 teaspoon hot sauce

DIRECTIONS

Soak the sweet potato in icy cold water for 30 minutes.

Drain the sweet potatoes and pat them dry with paper towels.

Toss the sweet potatoes with olive oil and salt.

Place in the lightly greased cooking basket.

Cook in the preheated Air Fryer at 360 degrees F for 14 minutes. Wok in batches.

While the sweet potatoes are cooking, make the spicy dip by whisking the remaining ingredients.

Place in the refrigerator until ready to serve.

Enjoy!

The Best Calamari Appetizer

Prep + Cook Time: 20 minutes

6 Servings

INGREDIENTS

1 ½ pounds calamari tubes, cleaned, cut into rings

Sea salt and ground black pepper, to taste

2 tablespoons lemon juice

1 cup cornmeal

1 cup all-purpose flour

1 teaspoon paprika

1 egg, whisked

¼ cup buttermilk

DIRECTIONS

Preheat your Air Fryer to 390 degrees F.

Rinse the calamari and pat it dry.

Season with salt and black pepper.

Drizzle lemon juice all over the calamari.

Now, combine the cornmeal, flour, and paprika in a bowl; add the whisked egg and buttermilk.

Dredge the calamari in the egg/flour mixture.

Arrange them in the cooking basket.

Spritz with cooking oil and cook for 9 to 12 minutes, shaking the basket occasionally.

Work in batches.

Serve with toothpicks.

Enjoy!

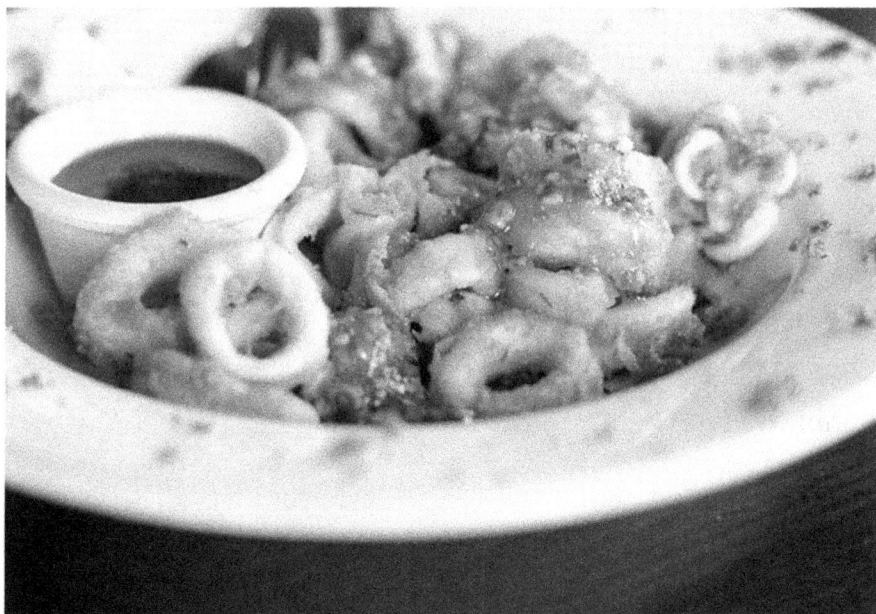

The Best Party Mix Ever

Prep + Cook Time: 15 minutes

10 Servings

INGREDIENTS

2 cups mini pretzels

1 cup mini crackers

1 cup peanuts

1 tablespoon Creole seasoning

2 tablespoons butter, melted

DIRECTIONS

Toss all ingredients in the Air Fryer basket.

Cook in the preheated Air Fryer at 360 degrees F approximately 9 minutes until lightly toasted.

Shake the basket periodically.

Enjoy!

Cocktail Sausage and Veggies on a Stick

Prep + Cook Time: 25 minutes

6 Servings

INGREDIENTS

16 cocktail sausages, halved

16 pearl onions

1 red bell pepper, cut into 1 ½-inch pieces

1 green bell pepper, cut into 1 ½-inch pieces

Salt and cracked black pepper, to taste

½ cup tomato chili sauce

Directions

Thread the cocktail sausages, pearl onions, and peppers alternately onto skewers.

Sprinkle with salt and black pepper.

Cook in the preheated Air Fryer at 380 degrees for 15 minutes, turning the skewers over once or twice to ensure even cooking.

Serve with the tomato chili sauce on the side. Enjoy!

Red Beet Chips with Pizza Sauce

Prep + Cook Time: 30 minutes

4 Servings

INGREDIENTS

1 red beets, thinly sliced

1 tablespoon grapeseed oil

1 teaspoon seasoned salt

½ teaspoon ground black pepper

¼ teaspoon cumin powder

½ cup pizza sauce

DIRECTIONS

Toss the red beets with the oil, salt, black pepper, and cumin powder.

Arrange the beet slices in a single layer in the Air Fryer basket.

Cook in the preheated Air Fryer at 330 degrees F for 13 minutes.

Serve with the pizza sauce and enjoy!

Fried Pickle Chips with Greek Yogurt Dip

Prep + Cook Time: 20 minutes

5 Servings

INGREDIENTS

½ cup cornmeal

½ cup all-purpose flour

1 teaspoon cayenne pepper

½ teaspoon shallot powder

1 teaspoon garlic powder

½ teaspoon porcini powder

Kosher salt and ground black pepper, to taste

2 eggs

2 cups pickle chips, pat dry with kitchen towels

Greek Yogurt Dip:

½ cup Greek yogurt

1 clove garlic, minced

¼ teaspoon ground black pepper

1 tablespoon fresh chives, chopped

DIRECTIONS

In a shallow bowl, mix the cornmeal and flour; add the seasonings and mix to combine well.

Beat the eggs in a separate shallow bowl.

Dredge the pickle chips in the flour mixture, then, in the egg mixture.

Press the pickle chips into the flour mixture again, coating evenly.

Cook in the preheated Air Fryer at 400 degrees F for 5 minutes; shake the basket and cook for 5 minutes more.

Work in batches.

Meanwhile, mix all the sauce ingredients until well combined.

Serve the fried pickles with the Greek yogurt dip and enjoy.

Parmesan Squash Chips

Prep + Cook Time: 20 minutes

3 Servings

INGREDIENTS

¾ pound butternut squash, cut into thin rounds

½ cup Parmesan cheese, grated

Sea salt and ground black pepper, to taste

1 teaspoon butter

½ cup ketchup

1 teaspoon Sriracha sauce

DIRECTIONS

Toss the butternut squash with Parmesan cheese, salt, black pepper and butter.

Transfer the butternut squash rounds to the Air Fryer cooking basket.

Air Fryer at 400 degrees F for 12 minutes.

Shake the Air Fryer basket periodically to ensure even cooking.

Work with batches.

While the parmesan squash chips are baking, whisk the ketchup and sriracha and set it aside.

Serve the parmesan squash chips with Sriracha ketchup and enjoy!

Hot Paprika Bacon Deviled Eggs

Prep + Cook Time: 15 minutes

4 Servings

INGREDIENTS

4 eggs

2 ounces bacon bits

2 tablespoons mayonnaise

2 tablespoons cream cheese

1 teaspoon hot sauce

½ teaspoon garlic, minced

1 tablespoon pickle relish

½ teaspoon hot paprika

Salt and ground black pepper, to taste

DIRECTIONS

Place the wire rack in the Air Fryer basket and lower the eggs onto the rack.

Cook the eggs at 260 degrees F for 15 minutes.

Transfer the eggs to an ice-cold water bath to stop cooking.

Peel the eggs under cold running water; slice them into halves, separating the whites and yolks.

Mash the egg yolks; add in the remaining ingredients and stir to combine; spoon the yolk mixture into the egg whites.

Serve and enjoy!

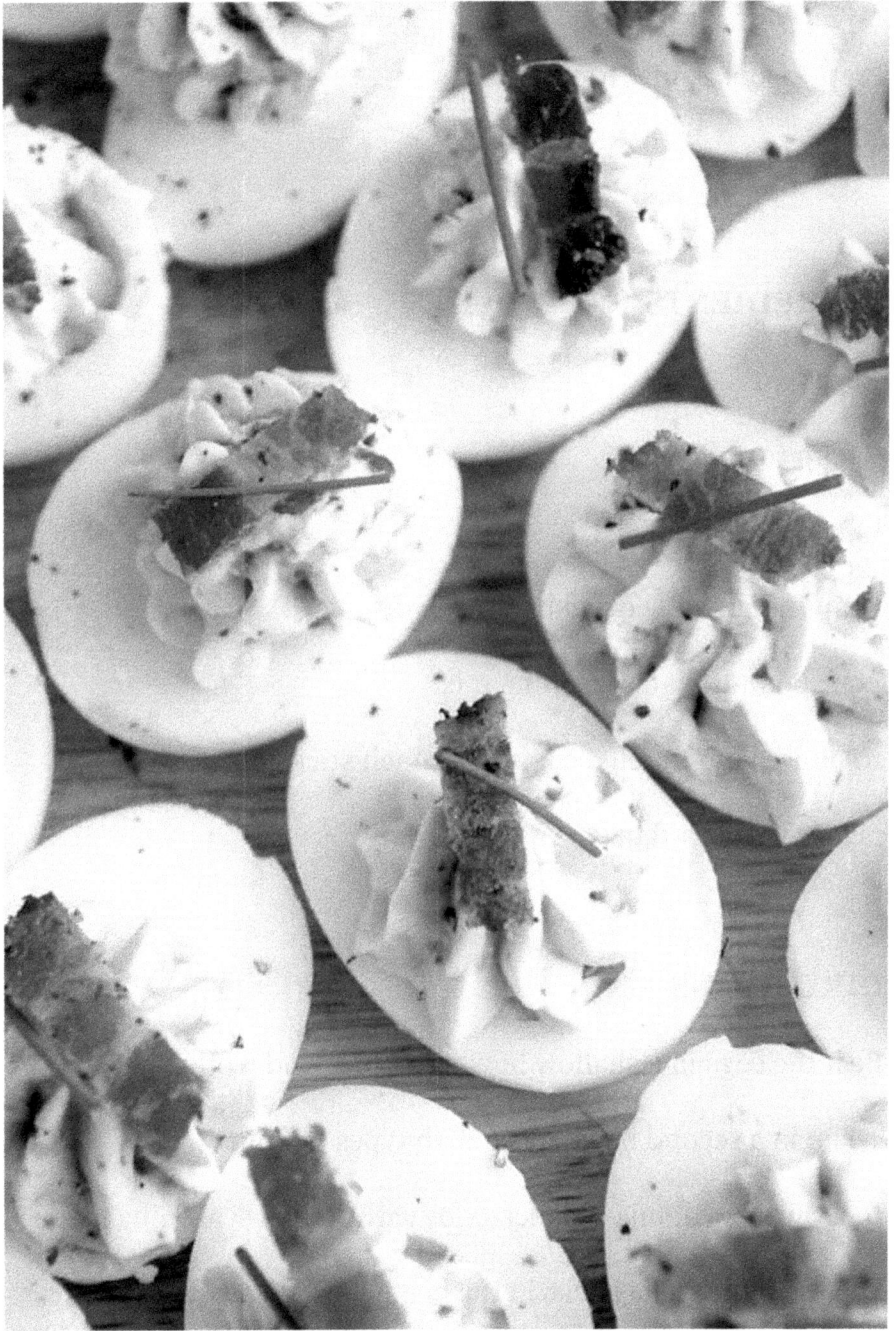

Kid-Friendly Mozzarella Sticks

Prep + Cook Time: 10 minutes

3 Servings

INGREDIENTS

2 eggs

¼ cup corn flour

¼ cup plain flour

1 cup Italian-style dried breadcrumbs

1 teaspoon Italian seasoning mix

10 ounces mozzarella, cut into ½-inch sticks

1 cup marinara sauce

DIRECTIONS

Beat the eggs in a shallow bowl until pale and frothy.

Then, in a second bowl, place both types of flour.

In a third bowl, mix breadcrumbs with Italian seasoning mix.

Dip the mozzarella sticks in the beaten eggs and allow the excess egg to drip back into the bowl.

Then, dip the mozzarella sticks in the flour mixture.

Lastly, roll them over the seasoned breadcrumbs.

Cook the mozzarella sticks in the preheated Air Fryer at 370 degrees F for 4 minutes.

Flip them over and continue to cook for 2 to 3 minutes more.

Serve the mozzarella sticks with marinara sauce.

Enjoy!

Famous Blooming Onion with Mayo Dip

Prep + Cook Time: 25 minutes

3 Servings

INGREDIENTS

1 large Vidalia onion

½ cup all-purpose flour

1 teaspoon salt

½ teaspoon ground black pepper

1 teaspoon cayenne pepper

½ teaspoon dried thyme

½ teaspoon dried oregano

½ teaspoon ground cumin

2 eggs

¼ cup milk

Mayo Dip:

3 tablespoons mayonnaise

3 tablespoons sour cream

1 tablespoon horseradish, drained

Kosher salt and freshly ground black pepper, to taste

DIRECTIONS

Cut off the top ½ inch of the Vidalia onion; peel your onion and place it cut-side down.

Starting ½ inch from the root, cut the onion in half.

Make a second cut that splits each half in two.

You will have 4 quarters held together by the root.

Repeat these cuts, splitting the 4 quarters to yield eighths; then, you should split them again until you have 16 evenly spaced cuts.

Turn the onion over and gently separate the outer pieces using your fingers.

In a mixing bowl, thoroughly combine the flour and spices.

In a separate bowl, whisk the eggs and milk.

Dip the onion into the egg mixture, followed by the flour mixture.

Spritz the onion with cooking spray and transfer to the lightly greased cooking basket.

Cook for 370 degrees F for 12 to 15 minutes.

Meanwhile, make the mayo dip by whisking the remaining ingredients.

Serve and enjoy!

Roasted Parsnip Sticks with Salted Caramel

Prep + Cook Time: 25 minutes

4 Servings

INGREDIENTS

1 pound parsnip, trimmed, scrubbed, cut into sticks

2 tablespoon avocado oil

2 tablespoons granulated sugar

2 tablespoons butter

¼ teaspoon ground allspice

½ teaspoon coarse salt

DIRECTIONS

Toss the parsnip with the avocado oil; bake in the preheated Air Fryer at 380 degrees F for 15 minutes, shaking the cooking basket occasionally to ensure even cooking.

Then, heat the sugar and 1 tablespoon of water in a small pan over medium heat.

Cook until the sugar has dissolved; bring to a boil.

Keep swirling the pan around until the sugar reaches a rich caramel color.

Pour in 2 tablespoons of cold water.

Now, add the butter, allspice, and salt.

The mixture should be runny.

Afterwards, drizzle the salted caramel over the roasted parsnip sticks and enjoy!

Sea Scallops and Bacon Skewers

Prep + Cook Time: 50 minutes

6 Servings

INGREDIENTS

½ pound sea scallops

½ cup coconut milk

6 ounces orange juice

1 tablespoon vermouth

Sea salt and ground black pepper, to taste

½ pound bacon, diced

1 shallot, diced

1 teaspoon garlic powder

1 teaspoon paprika

DIRECTIONS

In a ceramic bowl, place the sea scallops, coconut milk, orange juice, vermouth, salt, and black pepper; let it marinate for 30 minutes.

Assemble the skewers alternating the scallops, bacon, and shallots.

Sprinkle garlic powder and paprika all over the skewers.

Bake in the preheated air Fryer at 400 degrees F for 6 minutes.

Serve warm and enjoy!

Summer Meatball Skewers

Prep + Cook Time: 20 minutes

6 Servings

INGREDIENTS

½ pound ground pork

½ pound ground beef

1 teaspoon dried onion flakes

1 teaspoon fresh garlic, minced

1 teaspoon dried parsley flakes

Salt and black pepper, to taste

1 red pepper, 1-inch pieces

1 cup pearl onions

½ cup barbecue sauce

DIRECTIONS

Mix the ground meat with the onion flakes, garlic, parsley flakes, salt, and black pepper.

Shape the mixture into 1- inch balls.

Thread the meatballs, pearl onions, and peppers alternately onto skewers.

Microwave the barbecue sauce for 10 seconds.

Cook in the preheated Air Fryer at 380 degrees for 5 minutes.

Turn the skewers over halfway through the cooking time.

Brush with the sauce and cook for a further 5 minutes.

Work in batches.

Serve with the remaining barbecue sauce and enjoy!

Chicken Nuggets with Campfire Sauce

Prep + Cook Time: 20 minutes

6 Servings

INGREDIENTS

1 pound chicken breasts, slice into tenders

½ teaspoon cayenne pepper

Salt and black pepper, to taste

¼ cup cornmeal

1 egg, whisked

½ cup seasoned breadcrumbs

¼ cup mayo

¼ cup barbecue sauce

DIRECTIONS

Pat the chicken tenders dry with a kitchen towel.

Season with the cayenne pepper, salt, and black pepper.

Dip the chicken tenders into the cornmeal, followed by the egg.

Press the chicken tenders into the breadcrumbs, coating evenly.

Place the chicken tenders in the lightly greased Air Fryer basket.

Cook at 360 degrees for 9 to 12 minutes, turning them over to cook evenly.

In a mixing bowl, thoroughly combine the mayonnaise with the barbecue sauce.

Serve the chicken nuggets with the sauce for dipping.

Enjoy!

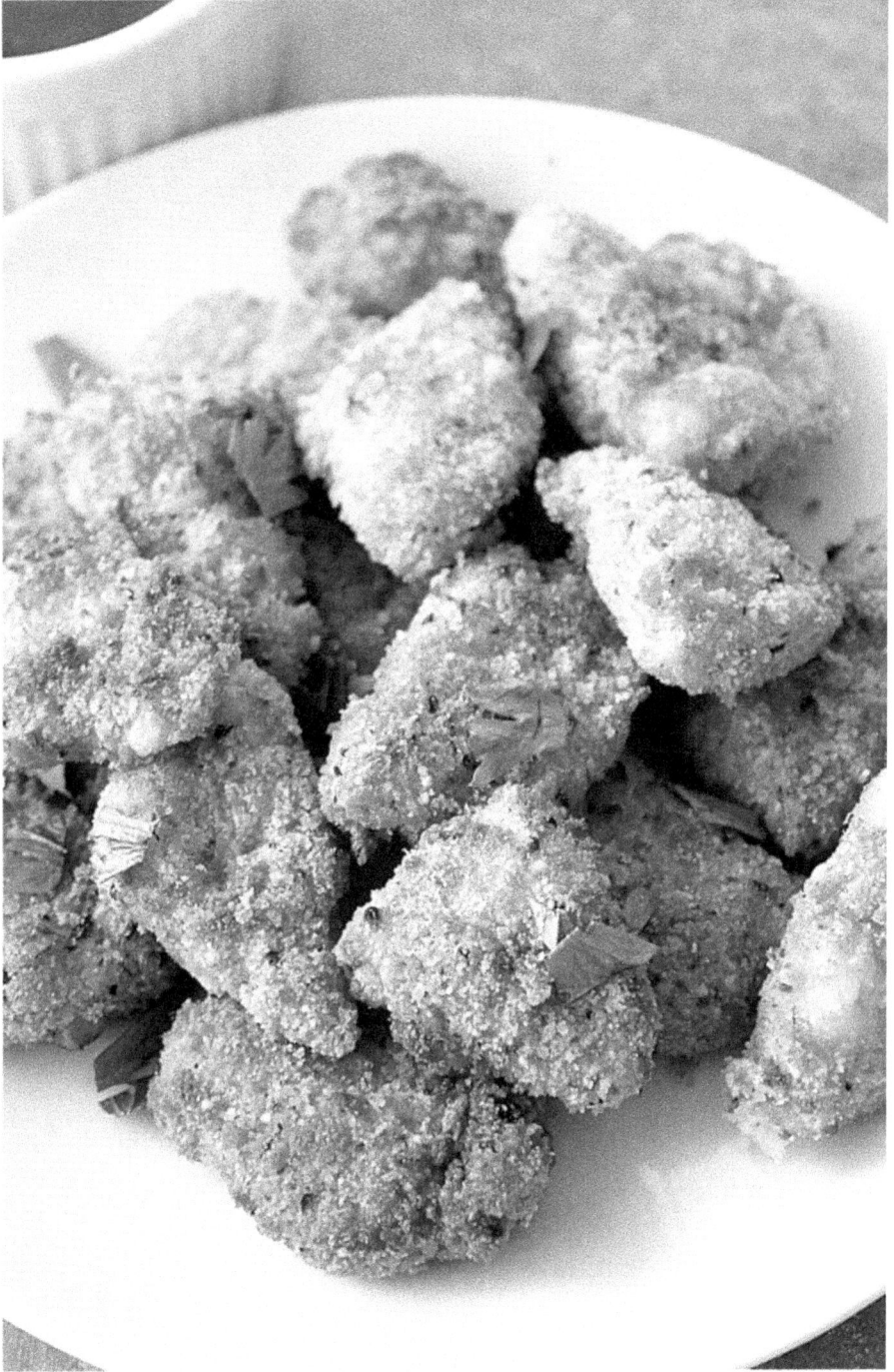

Sea Scallops and Bacon Kabobs

Prep + Cook Time: 10 minutes

2 Servings

INGREDIENTS

10 sea scallops, frozen

4 ounces bacon, diced

1 teaspoon garlic powder

1 teaspoon paprika

Sea salt and ground black pepper, to taste

DIRECTIONS

Assemble the skewers alternating sea scallops and bacon.

Sprinkle the garlic powder, paprika, salt and black pepper all over your kabobs.

Bake your kabobs in the preheated Air Fryer at 400 degrees F for 6 minutes.

Serve warm with your favorite sauce for dipping. Enjoy!

Chili-Lime French Fries

Prep + Cook Time: 20 minutes

3 Servings

INGREDIENTS

1 pound potatoes, peeled and cut into matchsticks

1 teaspoon olive oil

1 lime, freshly squeezed

1 teaspoon chili powder

Sea salt and ground black pepper, to taste

DIRECTIONS

Toss your potatoes with the remaining ingredients until well coated.

Transfer your potatoes to the Air Fryer cooking basket.

Cook the French fries at 370 degrees F for 9 minutes.

Shake the cooking basket and continue to cook for about 9 minutes.

Serve immediately. Enjoy!

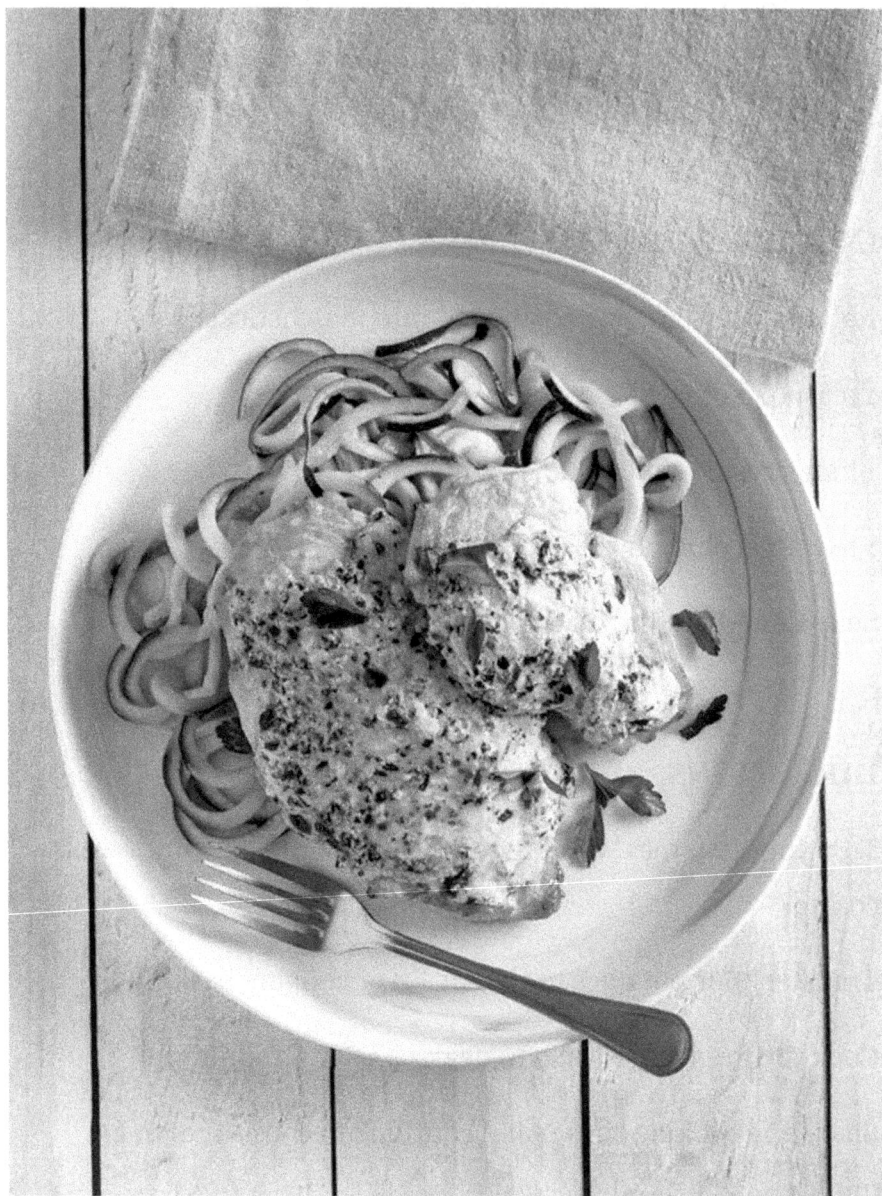